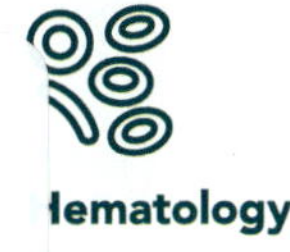

lematology

# First, the facts...

1. Beta thalassemia (BT) is a blood condition you're born with. It affects your red blood cells.

2. BT is a disease caused by changes (mutations) in genes that are passed on from parent to child. You have BT when you inherit a gene change from both of your parents.

3. There are two types of BT disease – BT major and BT intermedia. A person can also be a healthy carrier of BT without having the disease. This is called BT trait (or BT minor).

4. Treatment depends on the type of BT disease you have. People with BT major will require regular blood transfusions throughout their life.

5. New treatments for BT have recently been approved or are being tested in clinical trials around the world, with promising results.

**This booklet aims to help you understand BT so you can talk to your medical team about your condition and its treatment.**

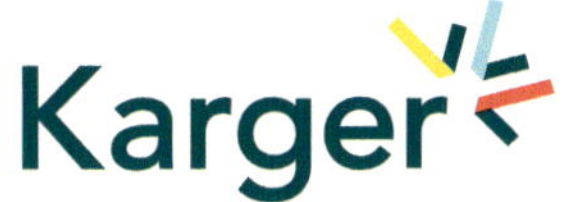

**HEALTHCARE**

# What is beta thalassemia?

Thalassemia is a condition you are born with. It affects **red blood cells**. There are two main types: alpha thalassemia and **beta thalassemia** (BT). This booklet is about BT.

In BT, the body doesn't make enough normal **hemoglobin** (Hb). Hb is the protein in red blood cells that enables them to carry oxygen around the body. There are also too few healthy red blood cells.

This is called **anemia**. Anemia can be mild or serious. Serious anemia can damage organs and can be fatal.

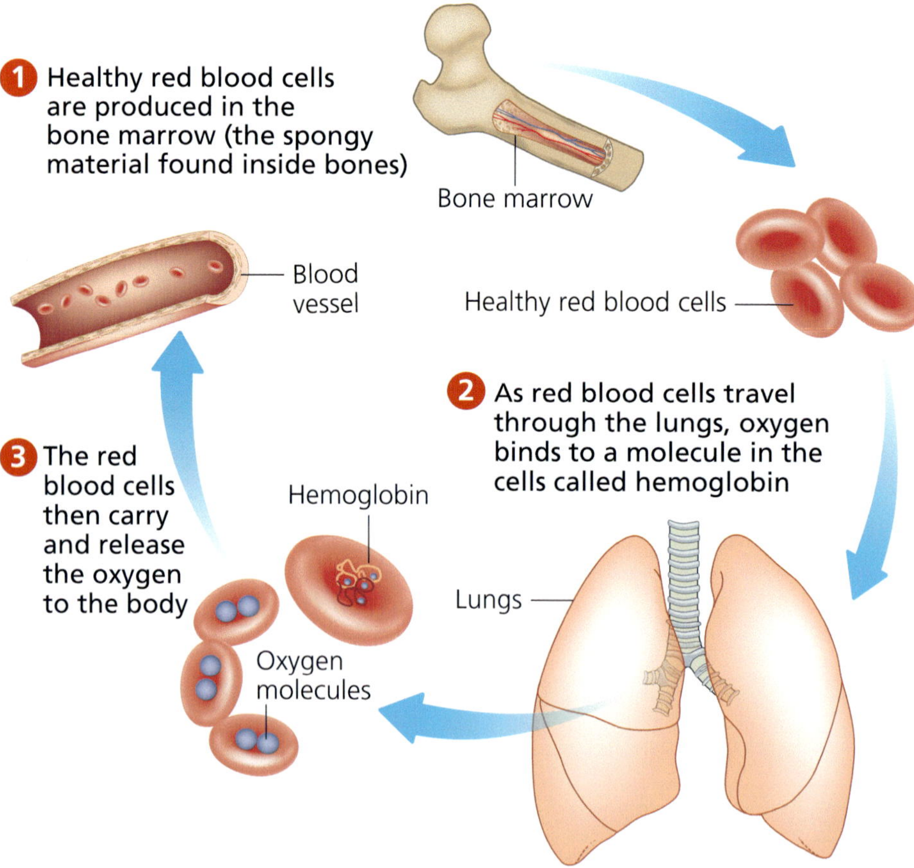

## Types of BT

There are different types of BT (see page 8). How severe your condition is and how bad your symptoms are depends on the type you have. You may have no symptoms, or you may need lifelong treatment.

## Why isn't the hemoglobin made properly?

Each molecule of normal adult Hb is made up of four protein chains – two alpha chains and two beta chains. If you have BT, your body is not producing enough of the beta chain. That means you cannot make enough normal Hb, so less oxygen can be carried around your body.

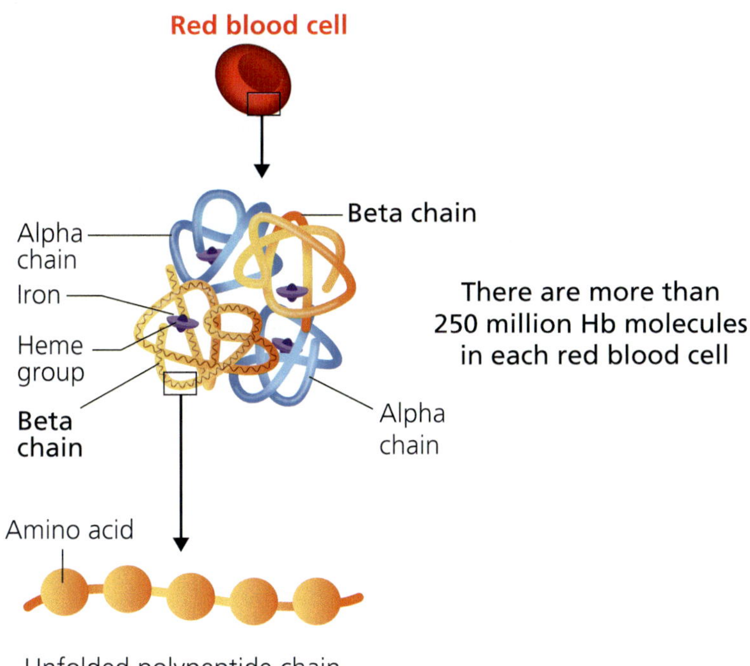

## What causes beta thalassemia?

BT is a **genetic condition**. This means it is caused by a change (also called a **mutation**) in a gene. There can be different types of change – some cause the beta chains of Hb to be missing completely, while others cause a decrease in beta chain production.

### What are genes?

Your **genes** carry instructions for the growth, development and function of your entire body.

Genes are found on **chromosomes**. Every cell in the human body has 23 pairs of chromosomes – so 46 chromosomes in total. Every chromosome has anywhere from 55 to 20 000 genes.

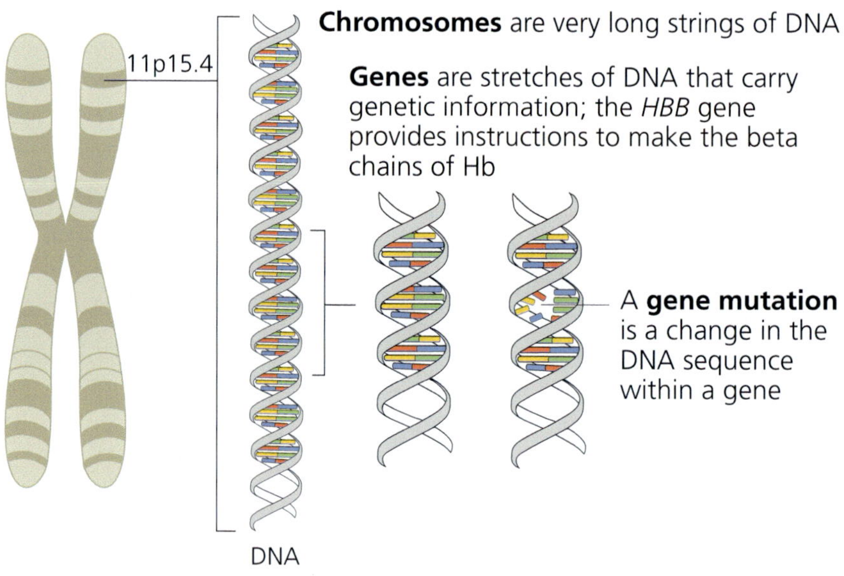

Genes are in pairs too – you inherit one copy from your mother and one copy from your father. A pair of genes is carried on a pair of chromosomes (one gene on each chromosome).

Each pair of genes carries the code to make a single protein.

The gene that carries the instructions for making the beta chain protein of Hb is called *HBB*.

## Who gets BT?

BT is more common in some parts of the world where malaria is, or has been, a problem (for example, the Mediterranean, the Middle East, North Africa, India and Southeast Asia) and in people with ancestry originating from these areas. This is because the gene changes that cause BT also give some protection against **malaria**.

Over time, the proportion of people in the population with a BT gene change has increased and, as people migrate around the world, BT has become more common in other regions too.

| My questions |
| --- |
| *Make a note about anything you want to ask your doctor here…* |

## Inheriting beta thalassemia

BT is nearly always a **recessive genetic condition**. In recessive conditions, both genes in a pair have to be affected to produce disease. This means you have to inherit a mutated gene from both of your parents to have the condition. So, either your parents have BT themselves, or, more commonly, they are 'carriers' of a mutated *HBB* gene.

**Carriers** have one mutated *HBB* gene and one healthy *HBB* gene. Because they have one healthy gene, they can still make enough healthy Hb beta chain protein. They will never develop BT, but they can pass on the mutated gene to their children.

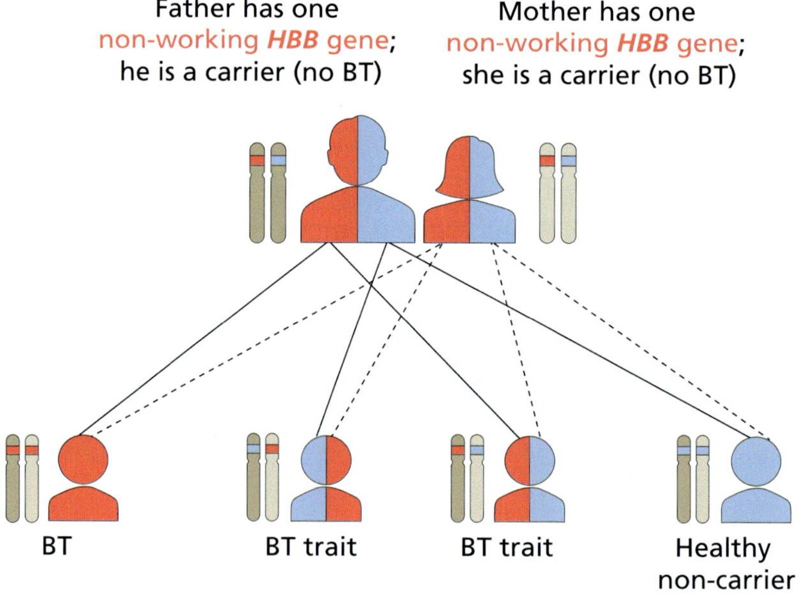


Being a carrier of a single mutated *HBB* gene is called **beta thalassemia trait** or **beta thalassemia minor**. There is a separate section about this and what it means for you on page 13.

## How do gene changes cause beta thalassemia?

There are many different changes to the *HBB* gene that can cause BT. How severely you are affected will depend on the type of gene change that you have. There are two main types of changes:

- Those that result in less beta chain protein than normal being made. Doctors write this as $\beta^+$.
- Those that result in no beta chain protein being made. Doctors write this as $\beta^0$.

Because there are two *HBB* genes, a person can have a combination of these types of change. You may have $\beta^+/\beta^+$, $\beta^+/\beta^0$ or $\beta^0/\beta^0$.

If only one gene of the pair is affected (BT trait), you may have $\beta^+/\beta$ or $\beta^0/\beta$. See page 13 for more about what this means.

There is another possible gene change, called HbE. This results in the production of an abnormal type of Hb known as hemoglobin E. So, you can also have the gene combinations $\beta^+/E^+$ or $\beta^0/E^+$.

**My gene change is...**

## Types of beta thalassemia

Symptoms of BT vary depending on which kind of gene change you have inherited. Because it's complex and to make things simpler, doctors generally put people with BT into two groups, regardless of the gene changes they have – people who depend on regular blood transfusions and those who don't. So, your BT may be described as **transfusion dependent** or **non-transfusion dependent**. People who need regular blood transfusions have more severe anemia (fewer healthy red blood cells).

**Commonly used words**

You may also hear the terms **beta thalassemia intermedia** and **beta thalassemia major**.

- BT intermedia (see page 15) describes less severe disease that does not need regular blood transfusions (although you may need more transfusions as you get older). It generally occurs when one or both gene changes are less severe.

- BT major describes severe disease since early childhood requiring lifelong regular blood transfusions. It generally results from a combination of two severe gene changes.

### Other types of inherited blood disorders

Sometimes people inherit a combination of a BT gene change and a change in a gene that causes another condition that affects Hb production. For example, some people have one BT gene change and the gene change that causes **sickle cell disease**: this combination causes a disease called sickle BT. Another condition is alpha gene triplication.

# Screening and diagnosis
## Newborn screening

In some parts of the world all newborn babies are screened for several genetic conditions. A nurse will prick the baby's heel with a fine needle and squeeze out a drop of blood, which is then used for the testing. The heel prick test is not a reliable test for all types of thalassemia but it can pick up BT major.

## Diagnostic testing

Children with the most severe forms of BT can develop symptoms from 3 months of age.

If your child has symptoms that suggest they may have BT, your doctor will request blood tests. These tests look for iron deficiency to rule out the commonest cause of anemia.

The blood tests will also analyze the Hb level, the shape and size of the red blood cells and look for changes in the structure of the Hb molecule. Carriers of a BT gene change and people with BT have red blood cells that are smaller than normal. This is a particular feature of BT called microcytosis. The specific test for BT is usually HPLC – high performance liquid chromatography – or sometimes electrophoresis.

**Commonly used words**

**Microcytosis** is the term used to describe red blood cells that are unusually small.

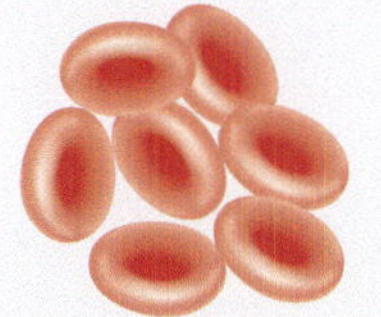

Normal red blood cells

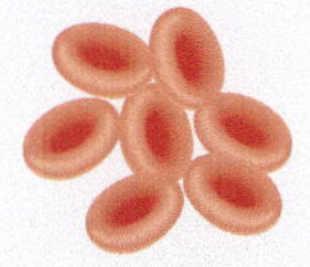

Microcytic red blood cells

## DNA tests

More than 400 gene changes are associated with BT. DNA (genetic) tests need to be done on a blood sample to identify the specific ones you have. The sample may need to be sent to a specialized laboratory for these tests.

### My questions

*Make a note about anything you want to ask your doctor here…*

## Pregnancy screening

Depending on your ethnic background or family history, your doctor may suggest you have blood tests for thalassemia if you are planning to start a family.

Ideally, tests for BT should be carried out before the start of pregnancy. But in practice, most women usually have blood tests when they first go to their doctor after becoming pregnant. If your blood test shows anemia and/or small red blood cells, your doctor is likely to suggest further testing for BT. If you are found to have BT trait (one changed gene), the baby's father will also need to be tested, to see if there is a risk your baby could be born with BT.

## Genetic counseling and pregnancy

If your doctor suspects you have a BT gene change, they may suggest genetic counseling for you and your partner. The counselor will help you understand why you are considered a 'couple at risk' for BT and will explain what your test results mean.

If the blood test results show there is a risk that your child could be born with BT, the counselor will continue to provide support. You will also be able to discuss your options when planning a pregnancy. Some couples opt to have in vitro fertilization (**IVF** or a test tube baby) so that genetic testing can be carried out before the fertilized egg is implanted. This makes sure that the baby doesn't have BT.

If you are already pregnant and there is a risk that the baby has BT, it's possible for the baby to be tested while still in the womb. This is usually done in one of two ways:
- taking a small sample of the placenta (chorionic villus sampling)
- testing the fluid surrounding the baby (amniocentesis).

Which test you have depends on how far through the pregnancy you are. Both tests carry a small risk of miscarriage, so your doctor will only suggest testing if absolutely necessary.

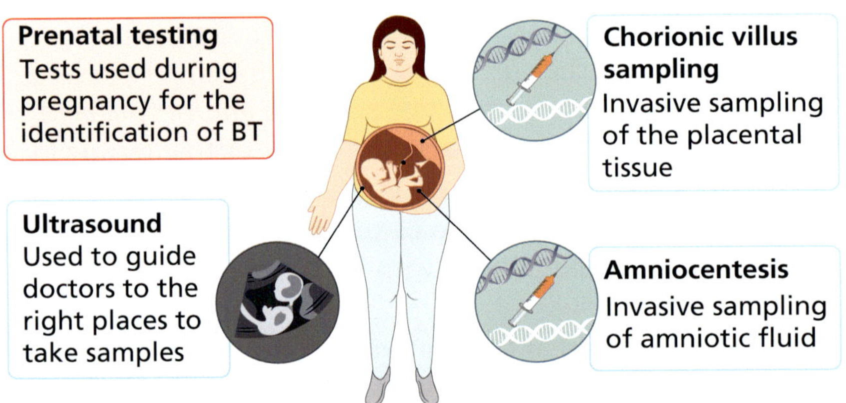


There are some non-invasive tests that are under investigation, such as testing fetal DNA found in the mother's bloodstream. These may be useful in future, but they are currently not accurate enough to use for thalassemia and give high levels of wrong results.

If tests suggest that a baby may be born with severe BT, your counselor may guide you through the difficult decision of whether to continue with the pregnancy. There is no single answer that suits every couple. The decision depends on lots of different factors, including cultural, social, spiritual and religious beliefs. Being fully informed about the disease will help you make a decision.

**Commonly used words**

**Invasive sampling** means a sample of tissue or fluid is taken from inside the body. This is done via a needle or a cut in the skin or through a body opening.

# Beta thalassemia trait

If you have only one changed *HBB* gene, you are a healthy carrier of BT but do not have, and will never develop, the disease. This is called **beta thalassemia trait** or **beta thalassemia minor**.

Normally BT trait doesn't cause symptoms so you may not know you have a BT gene change. A routine blood test may raise suspicions that you are a carrier but cannot prove this – you need to have specific DNA (genetic) tests carried out on a blood sample to find any thalassemia changes. BT carriers are healthy people who don't have thalassemia. You may have mild anemia, but this doesn't generally need treatment. You may have a pale complexion.

Under a microscope, your red blood cells will look small (microcytosis). A doctor who doesn't know your medical history may assume this is due to low iron, but it's not and you don't need iron supplements. In fact, you shouldn't take iron supplements unless a specific blood test shows that you are definitely deficient.

### What is the risk if I have children?

If you look back at the diagram on page 6, you'll see that if you carry a mutated *HBB* gene you have a 1 in 2 risk (50%) of passing it on to a child for each pregnancy that you conceive.

If your partner also has BT trait, there is a 1 in 4 chance (25%) of a baby having BT and a 1 in 4 chance (25%) of them not inheriting the gene mutation at all.

Your doctor may suggest you have genetic counseling if you have BT trait. There is more about this on page 11 in the section on **Screening and diagnosis**.

## What can I do to help myself?

You may feel tired if you have mild anemia, particularly if your body is under any extra strain, such as during pregnancy, or if you have an infection or have had surgery. You can help yourself to stay healthy by

- eating healthily
- exercising regularly
- not smoking or drinking too much alcohol.

## Should I tell other people?

When and how should you tell people that you are a thalassemia carrier? The simple answer is: whenever you are ready. Mostly, you don't have to tell people if you don't want to. But you particularly need to be open with your partner if you are thinking of starting a family in the future. They will need to be tested too.

Talking about a genetic problem can be difficult. People sometimes feel it's their fault. But you have no control over the genes you inherit. You can use this booklet to help others understand more about BT.

### My questions

*Make a note of any questions you have about how BT trait may affect you or your child here…*

# Beta thalassemia intermedia

Symptoms of BT intermedia can appear at any point. You may not need transfusions as it depends on the severity of your anemia and whether you need to prevent or control long-term complications. Your doctor will advise you about this.

## Signs and symptoms

You may:

- look pale
- lack energy when active or exercising
- not grow as much as expected
- not gain as much weight as expected
- have abdominal swelling, caused by the spleen getting bigger.

These may be the only symptoms if the condition is diagnosed early.

The spleen enlarges because one of its functions is to recycle and remove old and faulty red blood cells.

Symptoms can get worse when the body is under stress, because the need for oxygen is higher. Stress includes having an infection, recovering from surgery and during pregnancy.

### My questions

*Make a note of any questions you have about how BT intermedia may affect you or your child here...*

# Beta thalassemia major

BT major is a lifelong condition, with symptoms usually appearing during the first 2 years of life.

### Signs and symptoms

BT major causes severe signs and symptoms because the body is not able to make normal Hb. It is a transfusion-dependent condition.

Babies with BT major become thin and pale during their first year because of severe anemia. They also show early signs of bone changes (see page 17).

### Why is treatment important?

It's important for all children and adults with BT major to have treatment to control the disease and try to prevent complications as far as possible. If you don't, you are more likely to develop further problems as your body tries to cope with the faulty red blood cells.

There is more about these in the **Complications** section on page 17.

---

**My questions**

*Make a note of any questions you have about how BT major may affect you or your child here…*

---

# Complications

There are a number of complications that you may develop if you have BT. Some of these are the result of the disease itself, particularly if you don't have the treatment you need. Others are the result of a combination of the disease and its treatment.

### Bone changes

Children with BT major (and some with BT intermedia) who don't receive treatment may have bone deformities that develop slowly over time. The skull expands and heavy brows develop. Your doctor may call this **'bossing'**. The cheekbones get bigger, which alters the shape of the face, nose and eyes. It also affects the placement of the teeth.

'Bossing' does not mean that the bones become harder – in fact they are thinner and more fragile. Your doctor may call this **osteopenia** or **osteoporosis**. This increases the risk of fractures, mainly in the spine, ribs, pelvis and long bones.

**Commonly used words**

**Osteopenia** means that your bones have started to become thinner and more fragile. **Osteoporosis** means you have more severe bone thinning.

**Why do bone deformities occur?** Normally, blood cells are made inside the bones by a tissue called **bone marrow**. In BT there are fewer circulating red blood cells and less Hb than normal. To try to make up for this, the bone marrow becomes overactive and produces more and more red blood cells. But as these are abnormal, they die early and don't help to correct the anemia.

As the bone marrow continues to try to correct the anemia, it expands and this causes the bones to become bigger. It is this that causes the typical bone changes of BT. The more severe the form of BT, the more noticeable these changes will be. Treatment is with red blood cell transfusions.

## An enlarged spleen

Some people with BT major may also develop an enlarged liver (**hepatomegaly**) and spleen (**splenomegaly**), leading to abdominal swelling. This happens because the spleen removes faulty red blood cells and also because the liver and spleen become alternative sites for red blood cell production.

A very enlarged spleen can cause abdominal discomfort and make anemia worse. So, it may have to be removed.

Splenomegaly is more common and severe if you have non-transfusion-dependent BT. If you are having transfusions you will be receiving healthy normal red blood cells from donors and your spleen won't have to work so hard.

If you have BT trait, you may also have a slightly enlarged spleen, but not enough to cause symptoms.

## Gallstones

**Gallstones** can develop because of high levels of **bilirubin** in the liver caused by the chronic hemolysis. Hemolysis is the destruction of red blood cells.

If you have gallstones, you may feel bloated and sick (nauseated) and have abdominal pain. You may need surgery to have your gallbladder and the stones removed.

## Blood clots

There is an increased risk of blood clots (**thrombosis**) as you get older, particularly if you have non-transfusion-dependent BT. The risk is higher if you've had your spleen removed.

## Benign masses

Sometimes in BT, if the bone marrow isn't able to make enough blood cells, they can be made outside the bone marrow, in the liver and spleen. This can cause the liver and spleen to get bigger. But it can also cause small slow-growing lumps of tissue to develop, usually in the chest near the spine. These lumps (masses) are harmless but they can sometimes press on spinal nerves and cause problems. Although they are completely benign (not cancerous), doctors need to distinguish them from tumors on scans and X-rays and this can be difficult. Blood transfusions can prevent these from developing.

**Commonly used words**

When red blood cells are made in tissues other than the bone marrow, this is called **extramedullary erythropoiesis**. Common sites of extramedullary erythropoiesis include organs such as the liver and spleen, as well as lymphatic tissue, especially all along the spine.

**Leg ulcers**

Untreated BT intermedia can lead to problems with wound healing. Even minor wounds on the legs, particularly the ankles, don't heal and may get worse and become infected. These are treated with dressings to help them heal and antibiotics if infected.

# Iron-related complications

## Iron overload

Normally, when ageing red blood cells are broken down in the body, the iron that's released is recycled into new cells. When a person has regular blood transfusions, iron overload can also happen as donor red cells contain iron. Iron overload is when there is too much iron in your body. As the body can't get rid of all the extra iron, it builds up and can cause damage.

Iron overload can also develop in people who don't have regular transfusions (non-transfusion-dependent BT), but it develops more slowly. The buildup occurs because the overactive bone marrow sends signals to the gut to absorb much more iron from the diet. This happens because the body tries to correct the anemia by making more red blood cells and for this it needs iron.

Iron buildup can damage the liver, causing **fibrosis**. Fibrosis is scar tissue that replaces damaged liver tissue. If not controlled, fibrosis can develop into **cirrhosis** and liver failure.

Iron overload can also cause heart damage, leading to abnormal heart rhythms (arrhythmia) and eventually heart failure. Excess iron can also damage your bones and joints, increasing the risk of weakened bones (osteoporosis).

Hormone levels can be affected by iron overload too. Your thyroid hormone levels may be low, which can cause fatigue, weight gain and constipation.

You may be at a higher risk for diabetes. Iron affects the production of insulin in the pancreas, which controls blood sugar levels.

You may also have low levels of sex hormones. Puberty is often later than usual in children with BT. The low hormone levels may cause reduced fertility.

To help prevent all the problems caused by iron toxicity, your iron levels may need to be controlled with treatment called **chelation therapy**. Iron levels can be kept low and safe by the daily use of medicines called iron chelators.

See the **Treatment** section on page 23 for more about chelation therapy.

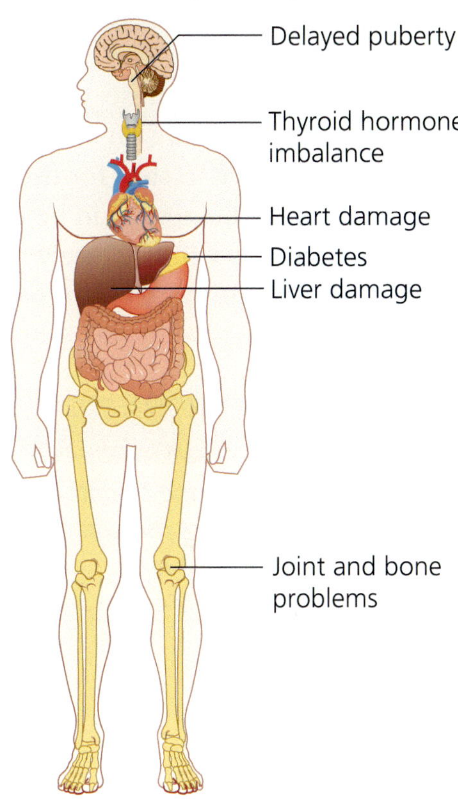

## Pregnancy-related complications

There are no particular complications from carrying a baby with BT. But if you have BT, pregnancy can put an extra strain on your body and make your symptoms worse. You may also have difficulty becoming pregnant, as iron overload can affect fertility (because of the effect on hormone levels).

You will need extra tests to check your heart, liver and bone health. If you are on **chelation therapy** (see page 25), you will have to stop for the first half of the pregnancy because the medicines could be toxic for the baby.

Your Hb levels will be closely monitored and you may need transfusions more often, particularly as the pregnancy progresses.

### My symptoms and complications

*Make a note of all the symptoms and complications you are experiencing so that you can make sure you discuss all of them with your doctor…*

*CONTD ...*

*CONTD ...*

# Treatment

BT is complex and needs specialist care. Your treatment should be managed at a specialist center for blood disorders and overseen by a doctor with experience in these diseases.

Specialist centers will often have a thalassemia clinical nurse specialist who you can contact if you have any queries when you're at home. Some centers also have psychologists and social workers who are familiar with the issues that BT can cause.

The two main treatments for BT are:

- **blood transfusions** to combat anemia and associated complications
- **chelation therapy** to control iron overload.

You may also receive:

- treatment for complications, such as an enlarged spleen and gallstones
- medication to improve the production of red blood cells
- stem cell transplant – an intensive treatment that is a potential cure for BT.

What treatment you have will depend on a number of things, including whether your BT is transfusion dependent or non-transfusion dependent.

### Non-transfusion-dependent beta thalassemia

You won't need regular **blood transfusions** if your bone marrow is making enough Hb for you to have a good quality of life and a low risk of disease-related complications. But this can change with time. As you get older, you may need to have transfusions more often. With any added physical stress, such as infection or pregnancy, you are also more likely to need a top-up of red blood cells from a transfusion.

Iron can build up in your body even if you don't have regular transfusions (see page 20). Your doctor will monitor your iron levels and treat any overload as necessary. There is more about this on page 25 (chelation therapy).

## Transfusion-dependent beta thalassemia

If your BT is transfusion dependent, you need lifelong treatment with blood transfusions to correct serious anemia and prevent disease-related complications. You will also need chelation therapy to keep your iron levels within safe limits. Having this treatment regularly is vital for preventing complications and ensuring normal growth, development and lifespan.

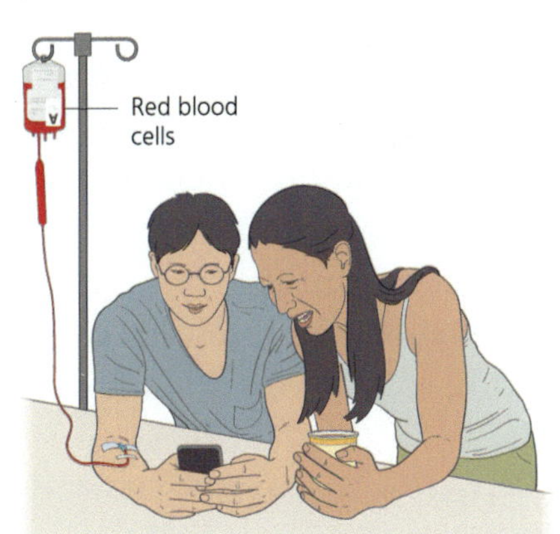


If your spleen becomes enlarged and hyperactive, your doctor may suggest removing it. But they will try to avoid surgery if at all possible. There are important long-term side effects associated with removing your spleen.

Stem cell transplant is now a possible cure for BT. But it is very intensive treatment and is only considered for BT major. There is more about stem cell transplants on page 28.

## Blood transfusions

Blood transfusions top up your levels of normal healthy Hb. How often you need blood transfusions will depend on your Hb level. Your doctors will want to keep this high enough to:

- prevent severe anemia
- allow normal growth and development
- prevent the bone changes associated with BT (see page 17).

If you have transfusion-dependent BT, you may need blood as often as every 2–4 weeks. The number of units of blood you will need depends on your body size. Your Hb level is a better guide for your treatment than the time since your last transfusion.

The blood you receive is carefully matched specifically for you, so that you don't have a reaction to the donor's red cells.

## Chelation therapy

As explained in the iron overload section (page 20), iron can build up in your body if you have BT. Too much iron is toxic so you will need iron chelation therapy to remove it.

Your doctor will monitor your iron levels with regular blood tests. If your levels seem high, you may have an **MRI scan** to measure the iron concentration in your heart and liver. This will show whether you need to start chelation therapy.

If you have regular transfusions for your BT, you'll need to start iron chelation therapy after you've had 10–20 units of blood. It is very important for your health to follow your doctor's instructions about iron chelation therapy.

| Chelating agent | Monitoring* | Considerations |
| --- | --- | --- |
| **Deferoxamine** (slow infusion under the skin [subcutaneous] or into a vein [intravenous] every day) | • Kidney and liver function tests<br>• Growth during childhood<br>• Hearing and eye tests | • Long infusion times every day can make it hard to stick to the treatment |
| **Deferasirox** (oral treatment once a day – tablets, a tablet mixed with water, or granules that can be sprinkled on food) | • Kidney and liver function tests<br>• Blood cell count<br>• Measurement of creatinine in the blood and protein in the urine<br>• Monitoring for signs of gastrointestinal ulcers and/or bleeding<br>• Hearing and eye tests | • The easiest for the patient, as the medication is swallowed or drunk once a day<br>• Risk of kidney disturbances |
| **Deferiprone** (oral treatment two or three times a day – tablets [USA only]) | • Blood cell count<br>• Liver function tests<br>• Measurement of zinc levels | • Risk of low white blood cell count |

*In addition to regular iron monitoring and/or MRI (magnetic resonance imaging: a type of body scan) to determine the amount of iron in the liver and heart.

Note: These drugs have other potential side effects, which should be discussed in detail with your BT healthcare team before starting treatment. The monitoring you receive may vary between treatment centers.

Your doctor will prescribe an iron chelating medicine for you. There are three different drugs available for chelation therapy. Two of them are available as oral medication and can be taken daily by mouth. One is a daily injection under the skin or it can be given through a drip (intravenous infusion or IVI). Sometimes, doctors prescribe two iron chelators in combination.

## My questions

*Make a note here of any questions you have about blood transfusions, chelation therapy or other treatments that you want to ask your doctor about …*

### Stem cell transplant

There is now a potential cure for BT, called **stem cell transplant** (SCT). This is intensive treatment that isn't available everywhere. Your doctor will carefully consider the decision to undertake SCT as the procedure has side effects, some of which can be life threatening. In the past SCT was reserved for younger children with BT. Today, young adults whose BT is well controlled are also considered for transplant.

Stem cells are cells in the bone marrow that are capable of developing into all the different types of blood cell, including red cells. In a transplant, the stem cells in your bone marrow are destroyed to make room for healthy cells from a donor. The donor has to be someone whose blood cells closely match yours, and this is usually a close family member. If you do not have a family member whose blood cells match yours, it is possible to search for an appropriate donor in bone marrow donor registries. Your doctor will need to find someone who is not related to you, but whose cells are a close match for yours.

The aim of SCT is that the donor stem cells will start to grow inside your bones and provide new blood stem cells to replace yours. This process is called 'engraftment'. The new stem cells will be able to make all the different types of blood cells you need, including healthy red cells.

The chemotherapy you have as part of your transplant increases your risk of infection. You will need to be nursed in complete isolation for some time after having your stem cell infusion. Other side effects of SCT include hair loss, sore mouth, sickness, diarrhea, bruising, bleeding and infertility.

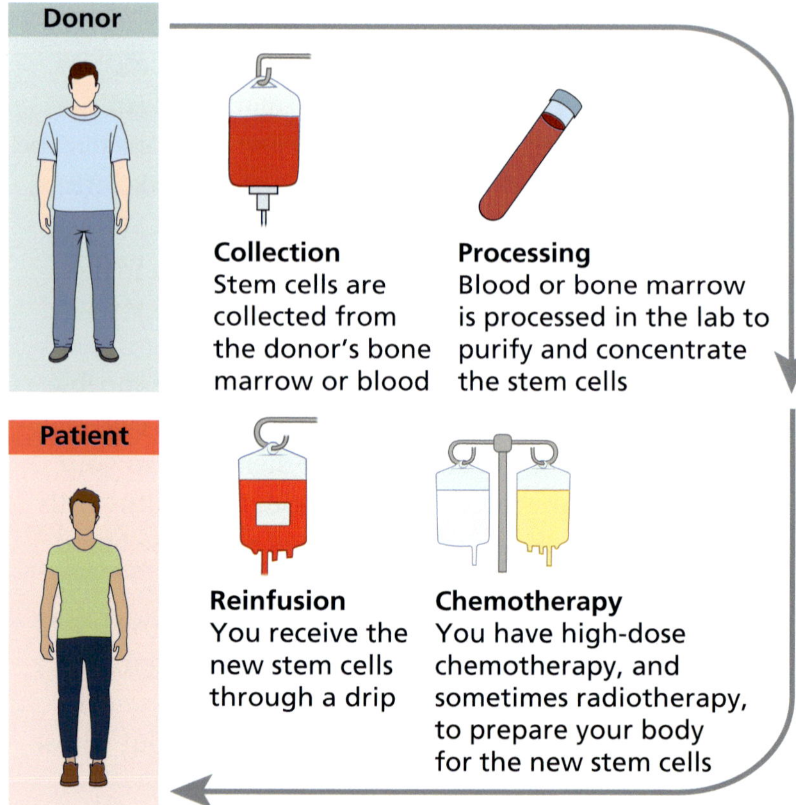



For some months after the procedure, you will need to take drugs to lower the activity of your immune system (this is called 'immunosuppression'). This reduces the risk of your own cells attacking the ones from your donor. Doctors call this 'rejection'.

## Stimulating the production of red blood cells

A medicine called luspatercept has been approved in Europe, the USA, Australia and many other countries, to treat adults with transfusion-dependent BT.

Luspatercept helps red blood cells to develop better in the bone marrow and so reduces the need for transfusions in BT. Some patients who were previously transfusion dependent may even be able to manage without further blood transfusions.

You have luspatercept as a small injection under the skin (subcutaneously) every 3 weeks. Some people have side effects, including headache and bone pain. Your doctor will be able to tell you if luspatercept is available and whether it is suitable for you.

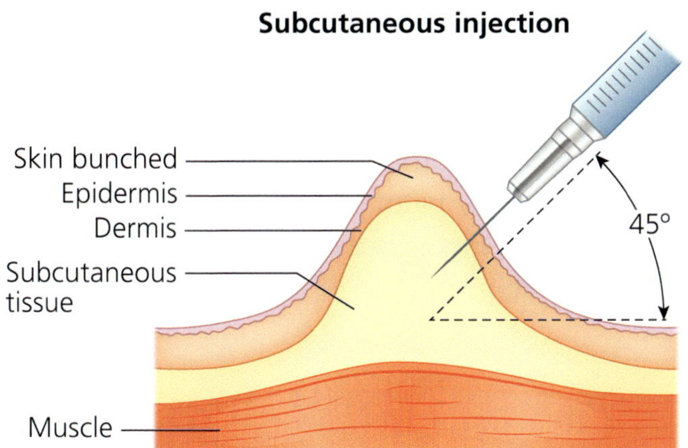



Luspatercept is now being investigated in clinical trials to see if it can help with non-transfusion-dependent BT and to see if it can be used in children.

# Treatment for complications

Some people need surgery for complications of BT, such as an enlarged spleen or gallstones.

## Enlarged spleen

A very enlarged spleen can cause abdominal discomfort and make anemia worse, so it may have to be removed. In BT, removing the spleen improves anemia and reduces the need for such frequent blood transfusions in some people.

Because BT is now much better controlled with transfusions, fewer people develop a very enlarged spleen and so **splenectomy** (surgery to remove the spleen) isn't done as often. However, people with non-transfusion dependent thalassemia may also need a splenectomy, as their thalassemia isn't managed with transfusions.

Splenectomy is a major operation and will require a stay in hospital and you will need time to recover. You may have **open surgery** (one larger incision) or **laparoscopic surgery** (several small incisions). Laparoscopic surgery is sometimes called keyhole surgery or bandaid surgery. With keyhole surgery, your hospital stay is generally shorter and recovery from surgery is faster.

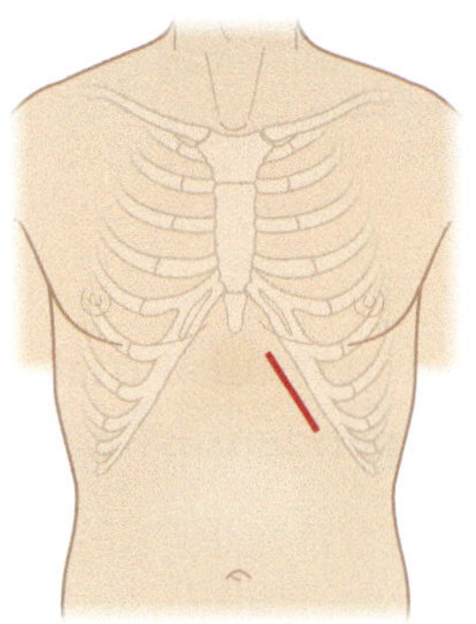

**Open splenectomy
incision site**

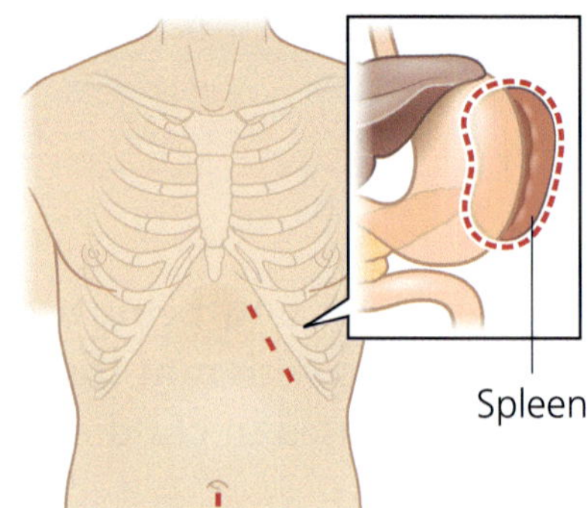


**Keyhole splenectomy
incision sites**

There can be other problems after you've had your spleen removed.

In BT, removing the spleen increases your risk of developing blood clots (**thrombosis**). This risk is lifelong and is the main reason why the benefits of surgery must be carefully weighed against the risks.

The spleen is part of your body's defense against infection so you are more at risk without it. To give you added protection, you will need some vaccinations, ideally before your surgery. If your child has their spleen removed, your doctor may also want them to take antibiotics daily for a couple of years after surgery to prevent infection. Or you may have an antibiotic prescription at home, so you can start taking them quickly if needed.

## Gallstones

Stones in your gallbladder can be very painful and make you feel very unwell.

The treatment is usually surgery to remove your gallbladder. You may have open surgery or keyhole surgery.

Keyhole surgery usually means a shorter stay in hospital and a quicker recovery as there is no large incision.

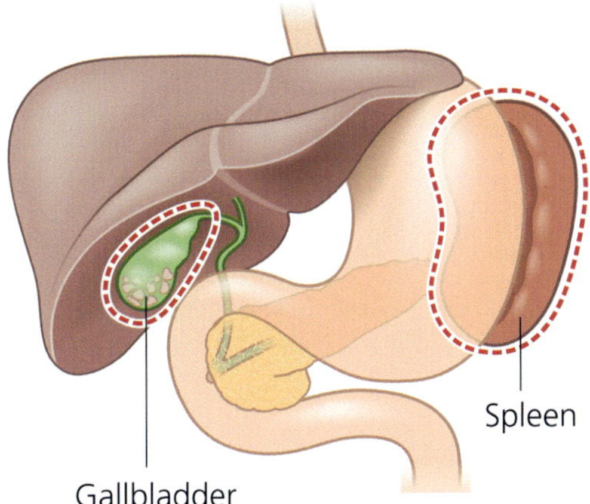

## Blood clots

People with BT may develop blood clots. The risk is higher in certain circumstances, such as before planned surgery, during pregnancy or after having your spleen removed. Your doctor may suggest you take medicines to reduce the risk of your blood clotting. You will have to have these if you've had your spleen removed. These medicines are called **anticoagulants** and include low-dose aspirin and heparin-like medicines.

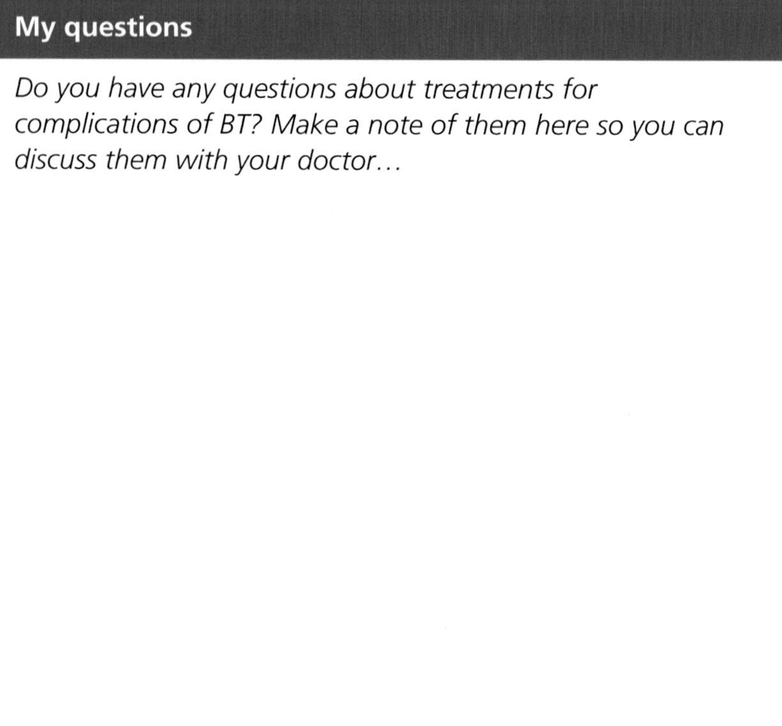

### My questions

*Do you have any questions about treatments for complications of BT? Make a note of them here so you can discuss them with your doctor…*

# New developments in treatment

If you are interested in new treatments, you may want to ask your doctor about **clinical trials**. A new treatment must go through several phases of testing before it can be proven to work better than existing treatment and be adopted into routine care. A potential treatment will only move on to the next phase of research if it is safe and shows promise.

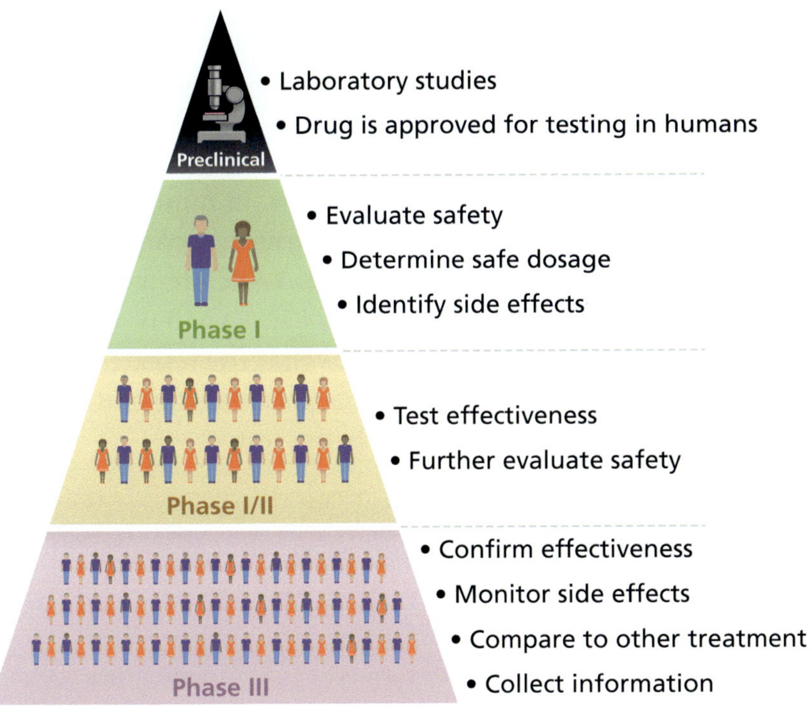

### Clinical trial phases

The first phase of testing – phase I – is to make sure a new treatment is safe, find out about its side effects and decide the best dosage. These trials are usually small, with only a few people in each one.

Phase II trials are larger and find out whether a new treatment is likely to work for a particular medical condition.

Phase III trials test the new treatment against the standard existing treatment to see which works best. These are the largest trials and are often international, particularly for rare conditions.

Phase III trials have to be randomized. In randomized trials, patients are put into different groups. A computer is used to decide who is in which group. You cannot choose which group you are in and so some people will not take the new treatment. Randomizing means that the researchers can be more sure that differences in the results at the end of the trial are caused by the treatment being tested.

**My questions about clinical trials …**

# New treatments for beta thalassemia

There are a few new treatments being tested for BT:

- gene therapy
- treatment to improve red blood cell health and function
- treatment to reduce iron absorption.

## Gene therapy

This type of treatment is showing promising results in treating BT. Scientists take some of your own blood stem cells and insert a Hb gene into them in the laboratory. You then have treatment to destroy your bone marrow cells, before you have the engineered stem cells put back into your bloodstream through a drip.

The process is very similar to having a SCT from a donor, except that your own cells are used. This means the treatment is possible for people who don't have a donor.

Like having a SCT, gene therapy isn't easy treatment to get through. You need to have chemotherapy, with all the side effects that brings. However, after the procedure you won't have to take drugs to damp down your immune system as you've had your own blood stem cells and not cells from someone else. There is more about SCT in the **Treatment** section on page 28.

Several trials of gene therapy have been carried out in people with transfusion-dependent BT and other trials are continuing.

A gene therapy was approved in 2022 in the US for people with transfusion-dependent BT.

## Improving red blood cell health

Clinical trials are looking into treating anemia with medication to improve the health, function and survival of red blood cells. In BT, it may mean you don't need transfusions so often.

Mitapivat is a new treatment that is being tested in people with alpha thalassemia or BT. It's a tablet that you take twice a day. It's already used to treat another genetic condition, called pyruvate kinase deficiency.

Mitapivat increases the level of an enzyme that red blood cells need to function properly. This enzyme is low in thalassemic red blood cells.

Early trial results show that mitapivat may help to reduce anemia in people with BT who don't need regular blood transfusions. Side effects found so far include difficulty sleeping, headache and dizziness.

Mitapivat is being tested in phase III trials for people with BT who don't need regular transfusions, as well as those who do.

## Reducing iron absorption

Researchers have identified a natural body hormone called hepcidin that reduces the absorption of iron from the digestive system and helps regulate iron levels in the body. Early trials used drugs that mimic hepcidin. These showed positive effects on iron levels in BT and also on red blood cell production.

A more recent approach uses treatments that target the main regulators of hepcidin. The first clinical trials of these treatments are under way.

# Living with beta thalassemia

Getting a diagnosis of BT – whether for yourself or your child – can be a shock, even if you know BT is in your family background. You are likely to have a lot of questions. It's important to find out as much as you can about BT and about your own situation.

To do that, it's best to talk to a knowledgeable healthcare professional or use other trusted sources of information about BT. Genetic counseling can also help you to understand your condition and its implications.

It can be difficult to know which websites on BT are accurate and have up-to-date information. To help you, there is a list of useful websites on page 46.

BT is complicated so it's easy to get confused. It may help to write down a list of the things you need to know or questions you want to ask and take it to your doctor's appointment. It may also help to take someone with you, so you can compare notes afterwards.

Treatment is improving all the time for BT. Many children born with the condition are now expected to have a normal life span, and there are things you can do to help yourself stay as healthy as possible.

## Have treatment when you need it

The best way to avoid complications is to stick to any treatment schedules and go to all your check-up appointments.

**IMPORTANT:** Contact your doctor promptly if you have any signs of infection or other illness and make sure you keep your vaccinations up to date – especially if you've had your spleen removed.

## Your diet

When you have thalassemia you may have low levels of some vitamins and minerals, such as vitamin C, zinc, **folic acid** and vitamin D. This is partly because of the anemia and partly because of high iron levels and the treatment used to remove iron. Your doctor may check your levels and give you supplements of anything that you're lacking.

Some doctors suggest avoiding foods that contain lots of iron and some think that this has little effect in preventing iron overload. It may be useful to check the iron content of packaged foods and medications and, in case of doubt, ask your healthcare team for advice.

It's always best to discuss your diet with your BT healthcare team.

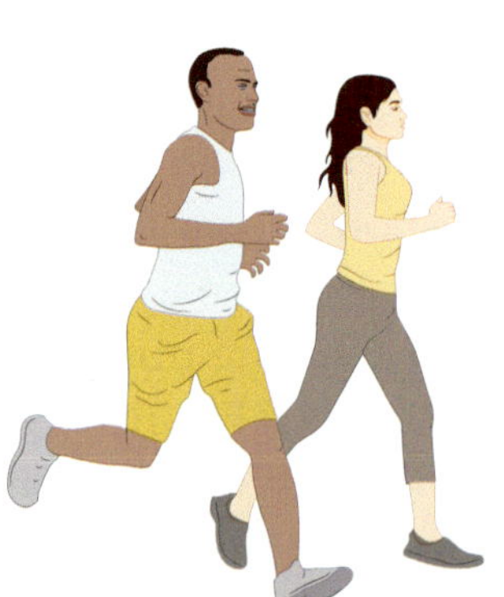

## Keep fit for healthy bones

Regular physical exercise has many benefits. It can improve your mood and help strengthen your bones. Alcohol and smoking are best avoided.

# Asking for help

Do ask questions and tell your healthcare team about anything that's concerning you. They know how complex BT is and won't mind, even if you ask the same questions more than once.

**Questions for your doctor**

*I've been told I'm a carrier of a BT gene – what are the implications for me and for my children?*

*What is the likelihood of me having a/another child with BT?*

*Is there anything that can be done to reduce the risk of having a child with BT?*

*What type of BT do I/does my child have?*

*What impact will BT have on me/my child?*

*Are there any particular warning signs I need to be aware of at home?*

*Will I/they need regular treatment?*

*Will my/their need for treatment change as I/they get older?*

*What are the likely side effects of treatment?*

*What complications could there be and how likely are they?*

*Will my child with BT be able to have children and what do they need to know beforehand?*

**You can record the names and contact details of your doctors, nurses and other support staff here**

*Name* ........................................................................................

*Role* ........................................................................................

*Phone* ......................................................................................

*Email* .......................................................................................


*Name* ........................................................................................

*Role* ........................................................................................

*Phone* ......................................................................................

*Email* .......................................................................................


*Name* ........................................................................................

*Role* ........................................................................................

*Phone* ......................................................................................

*Email* .......................................................................................

# Guide to words and phrases

**Alpha chain.** A type of protein chain needed to make normal adult hemoglobin.

**Anemia.** A shortage of healthy red blood cells, which can cause symptoms of fatigue and breathlessness.

**Anticoagulants.** Medicines that reduce blood clotting.

**Beta chain.** A type of protein chain that combines with alpha chains to make normal adult hemoglobin. Can be reduced or missing in people with BT.

**Beta thalassemia intermedia.** A type of beta thalassemia where some beta chains are made. At diagnosis BT intermedia is non-transfusion dependent, but over time it may become transfusion dependent.

**Beta thalassemia major.** A severe type of BT where no beta chains are made. BT major is always transfusion dependent.

**Beta thalassemia minor.** Now called BT trait.

**Bilirubin.** A pigment produced when old and damaged red blood cells are destroyed.

**Blood transfusion.** Receiving compatible donated blood through a drip (intravenous infusion) directly into your bloodstream.

**Bone marrow.** Spongy substance in the center of bones where blood cells are made.

**Bossing.** Abnormal bone growth in the skull, common in undertreated severe BT. Results in a large forehead and heavy cheekbones.

**BT trait.** Having one changed gene out of the two that code for the beta chain of hemoglobin. You don't have BT but you can pass the changed gene on to your children.

**Carrier.** Someone who carries and can pass on a gene change associated with a disease but does not have the disease themselves.

**Chelation therapy.** Treatment used to remove excess metals from the body – in the case of BT this is iron.

**Chromosome.** Long coiled strands of DNA. There are 23 pairs of chromosomes in human cells and one chromosome of each pair is inherited from each parent. Each chromosome contains many genes.

**Cirrhosis.** A liver disease caused by long-term liver damage. Healthy liver tissue is replaced with fibrous scar tissue and the liver shrinks and loses function.

**Clinical trial.** A research study to investigate a new test, treatment or medical procedure in people. Trials may look at whether a treatment is safe, its side effects, or how well a treatment works.

**DNA.** The genetic code that is the blueprint for how an organism develops and functions. Genes and chromosomes are made of DNA.

**Dominant gene mutation (change).** A person needs only one of the pair of genes to be mutated to have a condition or disease. Very rarely, BT can be caused by a dominant gene mutation.

**Extramedullary erythropoiesis.** The production of red blood cells in places other than the bone marrow.

**Ferritin.** A protein that stores iron inside your cells. As a blood test, it estimates the body's iron level.

**Fibrosis.** Thickening and stiffening of normal body tissues. Iron overload in BT can cause fibrosis of the liver and other tissues.

**Folic acid.** A B vitamin necessary for red blood cell production. Demand for folic acid increases when the bone marrow is overworked. Folic acid is often prescribed as a supplement for individuals with BT intermedia and sometimes for healthy carriers.

**Gallstones.** Hard lumps that can form in your gallbladder and cause pain and obstruction. In BT, they are caused by too much bilirubin.

**Gene.** Stretches of DNA that carry the codes for protein chains. They control growth and development of the body and are grouped together to form chromosomes.

**Genetic counseling.** A process that helps people to come to terms with having a genetic condition running in their family and understand their risk of passing on that condition to a child.

**Hb assessment.** The blood test used to look at the types and amounts of hemoglobin present in a blood sample.

**Hemoglobin A.** The prevalent adult hemoglobin in healthy people (normally >90%). It is made by 2 alpha and 2 beta chains.

**HbE.** An abnormal type of hemoglobin made by some people with BT.

**Hemoglobin.** The iron-containing protein in red blood cells that binds to oxygen and carries it throughout the body.

**Hepatomegaly.** An enlarged liver.

**Inheritance.** Passing genes onto your children.

**Iron-deficiency anemia.** A type of anemia caused by a lack of iron. BT is not caused by lack of iron.

**Iron overload.** A complication of BT where too much iron builds up in the body and causes damage.

**IVF.** Stands for in vitro fertilization. Also known as 'test tube baby'. A few eggs from a woman are fertilized outside the womb in the laboratory. This allows embryos to be screened for genetic conditions and the healthy one(s) to be implanted into the womb.

**Jaundice.** A yellowing of the skin and whites of the eyes caused by too much bilirubin in the body.

**Keyhole surgery.** Also called laparoscopic surgery or minimally invasive surgery. The operation is carried out through several small incisions, instead of one larger one. Recovery is often quicker.

**Malaria.** A serious disease caused by a parasite transmitted to people by mosquitos. The disease is milder in people who carry the gene change for thalassemia (BT trait).

**Microcytosis.** Means 'small cells'. People with BT trait have unusually small red cells, which can be confused with iron-deficiency anemia and other conditions.

**Mutation.** A change in a gene.

**Non-transfusion-dependent BT.** BT that is not severe enough to need regular blood transfusions. People with non-transfusion-dependent BT may develop transfusion-dependent BT as they get older.

**Open surgery.** Regular surgery, where the operation is carried out through a single large incision.

**Osteopenia.** Thinning of the bones that is not as severe as osteoporosis.

**Osteoporosis.** Thinning of the bones that weakens them and makes them prone to fracture.

**Protein.** A type of molecule made up of at least one polypeptide chain (a chain of amino acids.

**Recessive gene mutation (change).** If a condition is caused by a recessive gene change, both copies of the gene must have the change for a person to have the condition. BT is nearly always caused by recessive gene changes.

**Red blood cell.** A type of blood cell that contains hemoglobin and carries oxygen around the body.

**Screening.** The testing of a person or group of people for the presence of a disease or a condition such as a trait.

**Sickle cell disease.** Another genetic condition that affects red blood cells. Sometimes, people inherit one BT gene and one sickle cell gene, causing a disease called sickle BT.

**Spleen.** Body organ that is part of the immune system and responsible for destroying old and damaged red blood cells, for filtering them from the bloodstream and for destroying bacteria.

**Splenectomy.** Surgery to remove the spleen.

**Splenomegaly.** An enlarged spleen.

**Stem cell transplant.** An intensive treatment for some types of blood disorders. Can be a potential cure for BT.

**Thrombosis.** A blood clot.

**Transfusion-dependent BT.** Having BT severe enough to need regular blood transfusions. You may need transfusions throughout your life, or as you get older.

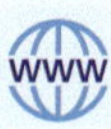

## Useful resources

**Northern California Comprehensive Thalassemia Center**
www.thalassemia.com

**Thalassaemia International Federation**
https://thalassaemia.org.cy

**UK Thalassaemia Society**
https://ukts.org

**Cooley's Anemia Foundation**
www.thalassemia.org

# Sources used in the preparation of this document

**BMJ Best Practice**
https://bestpractice.bmj.com

**British National Formulary**
https://bnf.nice.org.uk

**European Medicines Agency**
www.ema.europa.eu

**Medline Plus**
https://medlineplus.gov/

**Northern California Comprehensive Thalassemia Center**
https://thalassemia.com

**Royal College of Obstetrics and Gynaecology**
www.rcog.org.uk/globalassets/
documents/guidelines/
gtg_66_thalassaemia.pdf

**Thalassaemia International Federation**
https://thalassaemia.org.cy

**UK Thalassaemia Society**
https://ukts.org

**UpToDate**
www.wolterskluwer.com/en/
solutions/uptodate

Fast Facts for Patients

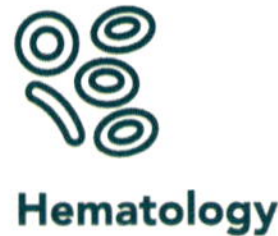

Hematology

**Antonio Piga MD, PhD**

Professor of Pediatrics, University of Turin, Italy

Medical writing support provided by Liz Woolf.

Made possible by a contribution from Agios. Agios did not have any influence on the content and all items were subject to independent and editorial review.

© 2023 in this edition, S. Karger Publishers Ltd.
ISBN: 978-3-318-07153-5

**We'd like your feedback**
How has this book helped you? Is there anything you didn't understand?
Do you still have any unanswered questions?
Please send your questions, or any other comments, to fastfacts@karger.com
and help readers of future editions. Thank you!

Quote from a young BT patient, made as a final comment after answering a questionnaire on quality of life…

*'If I could have the chance of a second life, I would choose to be thalassemic again, but I would ask for good care.'*

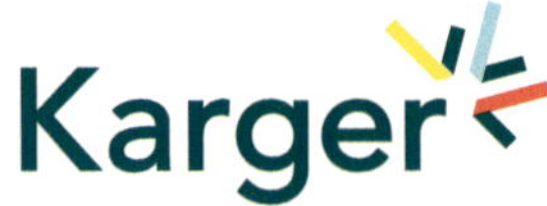

**HEALTHCARE**